# Study Guide for the
# Hospice and Palliative
# Nursing Assistant

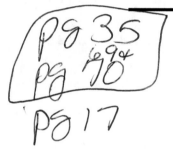

**Editor**
Barbara Anderson Head, RN, CHPN®, ACSW
Program Coordinator
University of Louisville School of Medicine
Louisville, KY

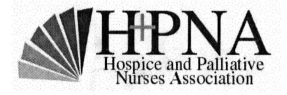

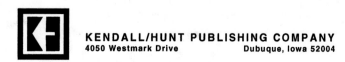

**KENDALL/HUNT PUBLISHING COMPANY**
4050 Westmark Drive          Dubuque, Iowa 52004

Development of this Study Guide

has been made possible by the

**Hospice and Palliative Nurses Association**

# Content Reviewers

Altha M. Barr
Certified Nursing Assistant
Hospice of Louisville
Louisville, KY

DeAnn King
Certified Nursing Assistant
Hospice of Louisville
Louisville, KY

Patricia M. LaVigna, CHPNA
Hospice of the Western Reserve
Cleveland, OH

Virginia Shubert, RN, MN
Executive Director
Yolo Hospice
Davis, CA

Susan Snider, RN, CHPN®, MSW
Associate Vice President of Nursing
Hospice of the Bluegrass
Lexington, KY

Margaret Fugate
Certified Nursing Assistant
Mountain Community Hospice
Hazard, KY

Jill Laird, RN, MN, CHPN®
Palliative Care Clinical Nurse Specialist
Virginia Commonwealth University Health System
Richmond, VA

Joanne E. Sheldon, MEd, RN, CHPN®
Education Coordinator
Hospice of the Western Reserve
Cleveland, OH

Rebecca Simpson, RN, BSN, CHPN®, CNA
Director of Clinical Services
Hospice and Palliative Care of Louisville
Louisville, KY

Chris Webb
Certified Nursing Assistant
Hospice of Louisville
Louisville, KY

# DISCLAIMER

The Hospice and Palliative Nurses Association, its officers and directors and the authors and reviewers of this Study Guide make no claims that buying or studying it will guarantee a passing score on the CHPNA Certification examination.

# CONTENTS

# CONTRIBUTORS

Brenda Kelly Burke, MS, APRN, BC
Professor of Nursing
New Hampshire Community
Technical College
Manchester, NY

Beth Miller Kraybill, RN, BSN, CHPN®
Research Nurse Coordinator
Swedish Medical Center
Seattle, WA

Marty Richards, MSW, ACSW, LICSW
Consultant
Gerontological Social Worker
Port Townsend, WA

Sarah Wilson, PhD, RN
Associate Professor
Marquette University
Milwaukee, WI

Eileen Chichin, PhD, RN
Co-Director
Greenberg Center on Ethics
New York, NY

Jayne Pawasauskas, PharmD, BCPS
Clinical Assistant Professor
University of Rhode Island
College of Pharmacology
Kingston, RI

Dena Jean Sutermaster, MSN, RN
Director of Education/Research
Hospice and Palliative Nurses Association
Pittsburgh, PA

# INTRODUCTION

HPNA recognizes the significant contribution to end-of-life care that is provided by nursing assistants. Nursing assistants provide much of the personal care needed by patients, spending more time with hospice and palliative patients than any other member of the team. To this end, HPNA is committed to developing educational products for the over 1000 nursing assistant HPNA members. In 2002, HPNA published the *Core Curriculum for the Hospice and Palliative Nursing Assistant.* Now, as an accompanying piece, HPNA has developed the *Study Guide for the Hospice and Palliative Nursing Assistant.*

The study guide is divided into two sections. The first section includes questions that cover the scope of the hospice and palliative nursing assistant in the areas of physical, spiritual, psychosocial and emotional care. The second section includes case studies that can be answered by an individual or used in a study group. Both the questions and case studies are followed by explanations of the answers.

This study guide is aimed at both experienced nursing assistants and nursing assistants new to hospice and palliative care. We welcome your feedback on whether this study guide meets your needs and if you have other ideas for educational product development for nursing assistants. We strive to provide useful and pertinent information to promote excellence in hospice and palliative care across all levels of nursing in all settings of care.

Constance Dahlin, MSN, APRN, BC-PCM
Vice President of the HPNA Board of Directors
Chair of HPNA Education/Research Committee
Clinical Nurse Specialist
Palliative Care Service
Massachusetts General Hospital
Boston, MA

# Editor's Comments

Those of us who work in hospice and palliative care are ever aware of the unique and valuable contribution of the nursing assistants who provide hands-on care and compassionate support to patients at the end of life. It is a very special person who can attend to the personal care needs of patients whose physical condition is declining while emotional and spiritual needs may be escalating. The job can be physically demanding and emotionally draining, but day after day these devoted care providers are at the bedside of those facing the challenges of terminal illness.

The hospice and palliative nursing assistant has a unique set of skills and expertise and the certification process delineates this work as a specialty—the first nursing specialty to offer a certification program. This certification process verifies and validates the knowledge of the nursing assistant and should be a source of great pride to both the individual who becomes certified and the employing organization.

It has indeed been an honor to assist with this project. My hope is that this guide will be a learning tool for nursing assistants preparing for the certification and will help build the confidence and knowledge needed for the process. Questions were developed based upon the *Core Curriculum for the Hospice and Palliative Nursing Assistant* and the test content outline developed by the National Board for Certification of Hospice and Palliative Nurses. Some questions may seem challenging, but the intent is to stimulate learning about the various content areas. This is only a guide for study and is not intended to reflect what the actual test for certification might include. Case studies (an approach not employed on the actual certification exam) are given for the purpose of exploring and thinking through situations common to hospice and palliative care.

Thanks to all the professionals who contributed questions to this guide and to the content reviewers who gave of their time and talent. I think I can speak for all of us in saying that we are very proud to contribute to the process of assuring that hospice and palliative nursing assistants receive the much deserved credit and affirmation for the skills and knowledge they have developed and utilize to make life's end one of comfort and meaning for their patients and families.

Barbara Anderson Head, RN, CHPN®, ACSW
Program Coordinator
University of Louisville School of Medicine
Louisville, KY

# Study Questions and Answers

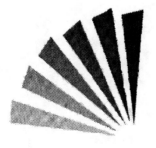

1. In providing support to a depressed patient, it is best to:

   A. Avoid discussing the past

   B. Try to cheer the patient

   C. Discourage independence and decision making

   D. Listen and allow the patient the time needed to respond and share feelings

2. In order to have a "good death" a patient must:

   A. Be a religious person

   B. Die at home

   C. Be free from avoidable pain and suffering

   D. Have medications available for sedation

3. Which of the following is **TRUE** about the end of life?

   A. It is the same for every patient

   B. It can be an opportunity for personal growth

   C. A good doctor can predict when the patient will die

   D. It usually happens suddenly rather than gradually

4. Which of the following is an example of nerve pain? Pain:

   A. From arthritis

   B. That's described as deep or crampy

   C. From shingles

   D. From a broken bone

1. Answer is D

   A. Incorrect: Avoiding discussion of the past or upsetting issues is not helpful to the depressed patient.

   B. Incorrect: False efforts to make the patient cheerful are not helpful.

   C. Incorrect: Making decisions and taking charge of oneself would be helpful to the depressed patient.

   D. **Correct**: The patient needs opportunities to explore feelings and share experiences.

2. Answer is C

   A. Incorrect: A person can have values and feelings leading to a good death without being religious in the traditional sense.

   B. Incorrect: The setting of death is not as important as how the death is handled and whether the patient's wishes are honored.

   C. **Correct**: It should be the goal of the palliative care team to make every patient as comfortable as possible during the dying process.

   D. Incorrect: Dying patients may be alert and aware as long as they are comfortable. Some require little or no medication.

3. Answer is B

   A. Incorrect: The experience of dying is unique for every patient and is a very personal experience.

   B. **Correct**: Many people can experience a sense of healing and well-being at the end of life.

   C. Incorrect: It is often very difficult, if not impossible, to know how a patient will respond to an illness and how long they might live.

   D. Incorrect: Most patients die after a period of illness and gradual decline.

4. Answer is C

   A. Incorrect: Pain from arthritis is an example of stimulation of pain receptors in the tissues such as joints.

   B. Incorrect: Pain that is described as deep or crampy is usually tissue pain in the organs.

   C. **Correct**: Pain from shingles is a type of nerve pain.

   D. Incorrect: Pain from a broken bone occurs from pain receptors in the tissues.

5. Your dying patient tells you that he just cannot force himself to eat. His wife is worried that he is "starving to death." In response to the wife's concerns, you should:

   A. Encourage her to make large portions of her husband's favorite foods

   B. Instruct the patient to spend time in the kitchen, hoping the smells of food will increase his appetite

   C. Provide emotional support and assure her that loss of appetite is very common at the end of life

   D. Suggest she talk to the doctor about a feeding tube

6. Which of the following statements is **TRUE** about an individual's culture? Culture:

   A. Does not change throughout a person's life

   B. Is continually changing

   C. Is inherited

   D. Is the same for every member of a specific ethnic group

7. You are the hospice nursing assistant for Mrs. Adams, a woman who has lived in the nursing home for many years. Mrs. Adams is alert and well-oriented, but her physical condition continues to get worse. She has told the hospice team that she does not want to go to the hospital if she gets sicker. You talk about Mrs. Adam's feelings with Mary, her primary nursing assistant on the 3 to 11 shift. Mary tells you she thinks that Mrs. Adams must be made to go to the hospital if she gets sicker. What should you say to Mary?

   A. "We must respect a patient's right to make decisions about their treatment."

   B. "You are correct and Mrs. Adams must be made to go to the hospital."

   C. "The social worker should talk to Mrs. Adam's family and tell them to overrule Mrs. Adam's decision."

   D. "The doctor will make the decision when the time comes."

5. Answer is C

    A. Incorrect: It is most likely that the patient will eat very small portions of his favorite foods.

    B. Incorrect: Strong odors can increase nausea and the gag reflex making it more difficult to eat.

    C. **Correct**: It can be hard for family members when their loved one is no longer interested in food. Family members may experience the following emotions: worry that the patient is "starving"; feelings of rejection; feelings of loss at giving up mealtime. Reassurance and emotional support are important at this time.

    D. Incorrect: It is outside the role of the nursing assistant to suggest artificial feeding. Studies have shown that artificial nutrition and hydration rarely help the dying patient feel better or gain weight.

6. Answer is B

    A. Incorrect: Culture is continuously changing and evolving.

    B. **Correct**: Culture is dynamic and constantly changing.

    C. Incorrect: Culture is acquired and learned in our families.

    D. Incorrect: Culture varies among persons even if they belong to a specific ethnic group.

7. Answer is A

    A. **Correct**: The Patient Self-Determination Act is federal legislation making it the law in every state that patients have the right to make decisions about their own treatment. Even if the healthcare team does not agree with the decision, they must respect it.

    B. Incorrect: The principle of respect for autonomy, as well as the Patient Self-Determination Act require respect for patient's wishes.

    C. Incorrect: The wishes of patients must be respected. The team is responsible for educating and helping the family to respect the patient's wishes.

    D. Incorrect: The patient's wishes are the most important issue and override what the doctor might want.

8.   You work on the evening shift and are assigned to work with a 75-year-old man who calls out from his room and asks for help. He tells you that he is seeing angels and their hands are stretched out for him. You respond by:

A.  Telling him that you do not see any angels and that he should try to go back to sleep

B.  Ignoring his talk about angels and asking if you can make him some warm milk because you know that is his favorite

C.  Asking him to tell you more about what he is seeing and listening carefully

D.  Not saying anything about his vision and tell him he was having a bad dream

9.   Which of the following is **TRUE** about palliative care?

A.  It is very different from hospice care

B.  It focuses more on symptom management than on curing the disease

C.  It is only available to patients who are close to death

D.  It does not address the patient's psychosocial or spiritual concerns

10.  Which of the following side effects of pain medications is likely †
     taking the pain medication?

A.  Nausea and vomiting

B.  Constipation

C.  Lack of appetite

D.  Itching

8. Answer is C

    A. Incorrect: Persons at the end of life may have visions or dreams that are symbols of dying (like the angels). Discounting those devalues the person.

    B. Incorrect: Ignoring what he tells you shows no respect for his situation.

    C. **Correct**: Asking the person more about his angel vision may tell you what is going on for him in his dying process. It also affirms him and what is happening in his life.

    D. Incorrect: Telling him he had a bad dream does not show respect for his experience.

9. Answer is B

    A. Incorrect: Palliative care complements hospice care and is very similar in philosophy and goals.

    B. **Correct**: Palliative care focuses on pain and symptom management when the disease cannot be cured.

    C. Incorrect: Palliative care is part of the continuum of care and can begin long before death.

    D. Incorrect: Palliative care focuses on psychosocial and spiritual needs as well as pain and symptom management.

swer is B

    ncorrect: Nausea and vomiting can be distressing short-term effects of pain medicine but they do t occur routinely. When they do occur, they are likely to decrease after the first few days of treat- t.

    ct: Constipation is a common side effect of pain medication, it continues throughout treat- nd requires a bowel protocol to be in place.

    : Though it may occur, lack of appetite is not a typical long-term side effect of pain medi-

    hing is a distressing but less common side effect of pain medication.

11. Which of the following is **TRUE** about the philosophy of hospice and palliative care?

   A. The primary focus is on providing expert medical care to the patient

   B. The patient is the unit of care

   C. Care is provided only during the final weeks of life

   D. Care provides support for the caregivers including the patient's family and friends

12. Which of the following statements is **TRUE** about acetaminophen?

   A. It should never be used with other pain medications

   B. It has no side effects

   C. It may be used before other pain medications for mild pain

   D. It is the best pain medication for inflammation

13. You have been working with an 80-year-old woman in a nursing home whose husband of 60 years visits daily. As you walk into the room the husband yells at you, "No one in this place cares about my wife." You are shocked because she is, in fact, a person whom all staff likes. Your best response would be to:

   A. Walk out of the room without responding and tell your supervisor what has just occurred

   B. Remember that this man has been through a lot. Gently ask him what you might do at that moment

   C. Ignore what he is saying and take care of his wife as you have always done

   D. Respond by saying "That's wrong. We care about your wife a lot."

11. Answer is D

   A. Incorrect: The focus of palliative care is on not only medical but also on psychosocial and spiritual care (the care of the whole person).

   B. Incorrect: The patient **and** the family are the unit of care.

   C. Incorrect: Palliative care can start early in the illness.

   D. **Correct**: Care does include the patient's family, friends and significant others.

12. Answer is C

   A. Incorrect: Acetaminophen is often used in combination with other pain medications.

   B. Incorrect: Serious side effects such as liver and kidney failure can occur with high doses.

   C. **Correct**: Acetaminophen alone can be effective for mild pain.

   D. Incorrect: Non-steroidal anti-inflammatory medications, such as ibuprofen, are better for inflammation.

13. Answer is B

   A. Incorrect: You need to acknowledge that you have heard his concerns by responding in a caring manner.

   B. **Correct**: You may not be able to deal with all of the deep-seated feelings that caused this reaction, but you can offer to help him with the immediate need that has brought about this comment from him.

   C. Incorrect: Not acknowledging him as a person shows a lack of respect.

   D. Incorrect: When you react by being defensive you may not really hear the feelings behind his words.

14. You walk into your patient's room and she says, "I can't catch my breath!" The first thing you would do is to:

A. Call 911

B. Contact the nurse and request that oxygen be provided

C. Offer a soothing backrub

D. Make sure she is sitting upright

15. Mrs. B came to your nursing home after suffering a serious stroke. She is unable to move one side of her body and needs help with many activities. Her healthcare team talks to her about whether or not she would like a DNR (do not resuscitate) order written in her medical chart. She asks you what you think about this. Your best answer would be to say:

A. "If you agree to a DNR you will not get any more treatment."

B. "Only people who are dying need to have a DNR order."

C. "If you have a DNR order, you will get treatment to keep you comfortable. If your heartbeat and breathing stop, nothing will be done to restart them."

D. "The doctor should decide what has to be done when the time comes."

16. To understand the cultures of others you must first:

A. Be aware of other cultures and examine your own attitudes

B. Read many books on culture

C. Interact with people from many different cultures

D. Have many experiences in other cultural settings

14. Answer is D

A. Incorrect: The goals of palliative and/or hospice care are to manage symptoms effectively in order to avoid emergency interventions. Calling 911 will start a series of events that are unlikely to meet the comfort needs of the patient.

B. Incorrect: There are many causes of shortness of breath. Oxygen may or may not be helpful to your patient depending on the cause.

C. Incorrect: This intervention may provide comfort once the shortness of breath has eased, but is unlikely to be welcome during a breathless episode.

D. **Correct**: Your initial intervention is to ensure the patient is sitting upright in a chair or with the head of the bed elevated. Suggesting leaning forward slightly, or resting with arms on an over-bed table may also be helpful.

15. Answer is C

A. Incorrect: A DNR order only applies to a situation where heartbeat and breathing stop and there is no effort to restart them with CPR or other means.

B. Incorrect: Older people who are so frail that they have to live in nursing homes almost never survive resuscitation, so it is recommended that almost all nursing home residents have DNR orders.

C. **Correct**: A DNR order only applies to a situation where heartbeat and breathing stop and CPR is not done.

D. Incorrect: It is a good idea for the healthcare team to know in advance what the patient's wishes are regarding this situation.

16. Answer is A

A. **Correct**: The process begins by cultural awareness and looking at your own feelings and prejudices toward other cultures.

B. Incorrect: Developing culture knowledge is the second step in the process.

C. Incorrect: Getting to know people of other cultures is important, but you should first understand your own feelings.

D. Incorrect: Having experiences with other cultures will develop your understanding after you have taken the first step of knowing yourself.

17. Mrs. Anderson has arthritis in her hands. She is most likely to describe this pain as:

    A. Dull and aching

    B. Shock-like and radiating

    C. Deep and crampy

    D. Cold and tingling

18. Your patient begins talking about her religious beliefs and practices. In response to this you should:

    A. Tell her to wait and talk with the hospice chaplain about this

    B. Try to quickly change the subject because you are not trained in this area

    C. Listen and ask questions without making judgments about the patient's beliefs

    D. Use this opportunity to tell the patient about your religious beliefs

19. Which of the following are common feelings of family members who are dealing with a dying loved one?

    A. Sadness

    B. Anger

    C. Guilt

    D. All of the above

17. Answer is A

    A. **Correct**: Pain from arthritis is usually described as dull and aching.

    B. Incorrect: These words are usually used to describe nerve pain.

    C. Incorrect: These words are usually used to describe visceral or organ pain.

    D. Incorrect: Pain from a broken bone is a type of somatic pain.

18. Answer is C

    A. Incorrect: You might encourage her to talk further with the chaplain but you would not tell her to wait when you could be a supportive listener.

    B. Incorrect: You do not need special training in religious beliefs to be a supportive listener.

    C. **Correct**: Being a good listener, asking appropriate questions and accepting the patient's beliefs are all spiritual interventions that the nursing assistant can provide.

    D. Incorrect: Sharing personal beliefs could be viewed as judging beliefs or trying to change the patient's beliefs.

19. Answer is D

    A. Incorrect: All are correct.

    B. Incorrect: All are correct.

    C. Incorrect: All are correct.

    D. **Correct**: All three of the feelings (sadness, anger and guilt) are commonly observed in grieving families.

20. In the United States, end-of-life care reflects the values of the American culture and healthcare system. These values include:

A. People should not be told they have a terminal illness because it is too upsetting

B. Physicians should make all decisions about end-of-life care

C. The family should make all decisions about end-of-life care

D. People should be told the truth about their illness and make decisions about how they will live out their final days

21. In practicing "active listening" with a person you should:

A. Take what a patient says at face value even if you don't understand

B. Be patient and listen to understand

C. Try to get them to move along in what they are talking about because you have only a limited amount of time to listen to them

D. As a timesaver, think about the next person with whom you are going to work while you are listening

22. Which of the following statements is **TRUE** about non-drug or complementary interventions such as massage and music therapy:

A. Most require a trained professional to perform

B. Not appropriate in patients with severe pain

C. Family members can often be taught how to perform such interventions

D. The patient's attitude towards such therapy is not important

20. Answer is D

    A. Incorrect: Americans believe people should be told the truth about their illness.

    B. Incorrect: The individual should make decisions about healthcare including end-of-life care.

    C. Incorrect: Decisions should be made by the individual. The family may have some input, but Americans generally believe that the individual should decide.

    D. **Correct**: The U.S. culture values people being informed and making their own decisions about healthcare and the end of life.

21. Answer is B

    A. Incorrect: You should always try to understand what a person is trying to communicate.

    B. **Correct**: It may take a few moments, but being patient and listening to understand assists you to learn what the person is trying to say.

    C. Incorrect: Even though you have a limited amount of time for each person, use that time to listen to what they have to say.

    D. Incorrect: Each minute of time spent with a person should be concentrated on the needs of that individual.

22. Answer is C

    A. Incorrect: Acupuncture requires a trained professional to perform, but most other non-drug interventions can be performed by caregivers.

    B. Incorrect: Complementary therapies can be used to decrease any level of pain.

    C. **Correct**: Many of the non-drug interventions can be taught to family members, caregivers or friends of the patient.

    D. Incorrect: The patient's attitude about the intervention should be discussed and non-drug interventions should only be used with the patient's permission.

23. Which of the following statements is **NOT** true about non-steroidal anti-inflammatory drugs (NSAIDs) such as ibuprofen?

A. They are only useful for pain, not inflammation

B. Patients on NSAIDs should be monitored for bleeding

C. They can cause stomach upset

D. Side effects of NSAIDs are more common and serious in elderly patients

24. Which of the following is a sign or symptom that the patient is close to death:

A. Long pauses between breaths

B. Pink color in the hand and feet

C. Increased social interaction with family and staff

D. Increased amount of urine output

25. The role of the nursing assistant in pain management includes:

A. Recommending a different medication

B. Completing the patient's schedule of medications

C. Observing for the side effect of medications

D. Teaching the patient and family how to apply a transdermal pain patch

23. Answer is A

   A. **Correct**: NSAIDs are useful for both pain and inflammation.

   B. Incorrect: Gastrointestinal bleeding may occur in the patient on NSAIDS.

   C. Incorrect: Stomach upset is a common side effect of NSAIDS.

   D. Incorrect: Elderly patients are more likely to have serious side effects due to the effects of aging on how the body processes the medications.

24. Answer is A

   A. **Correct**: A breathing pattern that includes pauses and changes in rate (often referred to as Cheyne-Stokes breathing) is common in the final stages of life.

   B. Incorrect: As death nears, the heart and lungs work hard to supply the most important organs with blood, leaving less blood available for the distant parts of the body. Often the skin becomes blue-tinged or very pale.

   C. Incorrect: Decreased social interaction is common at the end of life. The dying person usually spends more time sleeping and limits social interactions when awake.

   D. Incorrect: Though urine incontinence is common at the end of life, it is usually small in amount and dark colored.

25. Answer is C

   A. Incorrect: You should report your observations to the licensed nurse who will discuss any changes with the physician.

   B. Incorrect: The licensed nurse should complete any schedule for medications.

   C. **Correct**: The nursing assistant should be aware of common side effects of pain medications and report any that occur to the team nurse.

   D. Incorrect: Again, this is the role of the licensed nurse.

26. Mr. James is very upset that his wife died while he had left to run a necessary errand. Your best response to him would be:

A. Allow him to express his feelings and provide emotional support

B. Blame the nurse for not telling him that Mrs. James was approaching death

C. Tell him that she wasn't aware she was alone when she died

D. Ask him why his daughter couldn't have run the errand for him

27. Nursing assistant interventions to help a family grieve as the patient dies would include:

A. Discussing the weather or news to help distract them from the sadness of the event

B. Avoiding any discussion of the patient's condition

C. Keeping them informed of the patient's status and what to expect

D. Crying with the family

28. Physical causes of restlessness in the patient who is dying can include all of the following **EXCEPT**:

A. A full bladder

B. Constipation and/or impaction

C. Lack of oxygen

D. Hunger

26.	Answer is A

    A.	**Correct**: Often patients die when family members have left. Mr. James needs reassurance that he did not neglect his wife by leaving.

    B.	Incorrect: No one ever knows when a patient will die and it is always inappropriate to blame another team member for a problem.

    C.	Incorrect: No one knows exactly what patients are aware of, even if they appear to be comatose or unconscious.

    D.	Incorrect: Asking such a question would only make Mr. James feel worse about the situation.

27.	Answer is C

    A.	Incorrect: It is inappropriate to act as if the patient's dying weren't the most important issue of the moment.

    B.	Incorrect: Again, it is inappropriate to ignore the importance of the situation by not discussing it.

    C.	**Correct**: Education and preparation help the family to work through their grief in a healthy manner.

    D.	Incorrect: While it is important to express your concern, crying with the family will not give them the emotional support they need to deal with their grief.

28.	Answer is D

    A.	Incorrect: A full bladder can be a cause of terminal restlessness.

    B.	Incorrect: Constipation and/or impaction can also cause terminal restlessness.

    C.	Incorrect: Lack of oxygen or hypoxia can cause confusion and restlessness.

    D.	**Correct**: Hunger in the dying patient is not known to cause restlessness or discomfort.

29. Which of the following actions would support a patient's sense of dignity?

   A. Making as many decisions as possible for the patient

   B. Whispering to others in the room about the patient

   C. Calling the patient by his or her first name or nickname

   D. Speaking directly to the patient even if he or she is unable to respond

30. The two major types of advance directives are:

   A. DNR orders and prescriptions

   B. CPR and DNR orders

   C. Living will and durable power of attorney for healthcare

   D. Funeral planning and wills

31. The most important thing to consider as the patient nears death is:

   A. The team's care plan for the patient

   B. The patient's most important needs and goals

   C. Proper positioning of the patient

   D. Keeping the patient clean and dry

29. Answer is D

   A. Incorrect: Allowing the patient as much control over their environment and caregiving is important to a patient's dignity.

   B. Incorrect: Avoid speaking or whispering as if the patient weren't present. The patient will feel left out and forgotten.

   C. Incorrect: It is more respectful to use the patient's formal name (for example, Mrs. Jones, Dr. Lewis) unless the patient instructs you otherwise.

   D. **Correct**: Always speak directly and clearly to the patient assuming that the patient can hear all conversations. No one really knows how much the patient can hear even when unconscious or unresponsive.

30. Answer is C

   A. Incorrect: These are orders given by the physician and have nothing to do with advance directives.

   B. Incorrect: These orders have to do with actions to take should the patient quit breathing.

   C. **Correct**: These two directives state the patient's wishes should he or she become unable to make decisions. The living will states the patient's desires related to treatment and the durable power of attorney for healthcare names a person to make decisions for the patient when and if the patient becomes unable to make healthcare decisions.

   D. Incorrect: While these are both types of plans patients can make, they are not considered advance directives.

31. Answer is B

   A. Incorrect: The team's plan is important, but the immediate needs and wishes of the patient take priority as death nears.

   B. **Correct**: The patient's wishes related to their death and their needs for comfort are most important.

   C. Incorrect: As death approaches, positioning for comfort is more important than correct positioning.

   D. Incorrect: While this is important, it is secondary to the patient's immediate needs and comfort.

32. Mrs. Jackson asks you to read from her prayer book. Your best response would be to:

    A. Tell her you are of a different faith and don't agree with her prayers

    B. Tell her you don't have time to read today

    C. Read to her from her prayer book as requested

    D. Tell her you will let the chaplain know of her request

33. You have arrived at Mr. Martin's home to find him very anxious, moving around the bed restlessly and saying, "Help me, help me!" Your first action is to:

    A. Thoroughly question the patient about what happened today to make him so nervous

    B. Restrain the patient and call the RN to report the problem

    C. Approach the patient in a calm and gentle manner and ask, "How can I help you?"

    D. Ask the family if the patient has medication for anxiety

32.   Answer is C

   A.  Incorrect: Your religious beliefs are not the issue here. As a member of the hospice team, your job is to help with the patient's spiritual needs.

   B.  Incorrect: You should always take time to respond to the needs and requests of the patient you are with at the time.

   C.  **Correct**: Reading to the patient from the prayer book assists with that patient's spiritual needs and desires.

   D.  Incorrect: While you should inform the chaplain of the patient's request and your response, as a member of the team, you can assist with this request and not put the patient off.

33.   Answer is C

   A.  Incorrect: Questioning the patient will only add to his anxiety.

   B.  Incorrect: Restraint is not appropriate unless all other means of calming the patient fail. While you should report the incident to the nurse, you should first attend to the patient.

   C.  **Correct**: A calm response that shows concern and understanding often settles the patient down and gets to the source of the problem.

   D.  Incorrect: Medication is a possible intervention, but supporting and assisting the patient should be the first response.

34. Your patient is dying on the hospice inpatient unit. The most important consideration related to the environment would be:

A. Maintaining clean conditions

B. Limiting visitors

C. Creating space that is comfortable and welcoming for the patient and family

D. Keeping the door closed at all times

35. Assisted death means:

A. Acting to end the life of a patient to relieve suffering

B. Giving patients strong medications to ease their pain

C. Providing a person with a medication knowing the patient intends to use it to commit suicide

D. A and C

36. Mrs. Black has had her pain well-controlled by medication, but when you visit her, she complains of terrible pain and rates her pain as 7 out of 10. However, she is sitting comfortably in her chair and does not appear to be in distress. In response, you:

A. Ask her husband if he thinks she is in pain

B. Make a note of this to report at the next team meeting

C. Tell her she doesn't look like she's in pain and ask what is really bothering her

D. Notify the RN immediately

34.    Answer is C

    A.  Incorrect: Clean conditions are important but not the most important consideration.

    B.  Incorrect: Unless disruptive and upsetting to the patient, visitors should not be limited.

    C.  **Correct**: The environment should be inviting and comforting and as homelike as possible.

    D.  Incorrect: Whether or not the door is closed depends on the patient's and family's preference and the impact on other patients in the unit.

35.    Answer is D

    A.  Incorrect: Although this is a correct answer, C is also correct therefore the correct answer choice for this question would be D.

    B.  Incorrect: While strong pain medications may seem to contribute to a patient's death, they are given to relieve the patient's pain and not to hasten the patient's death.

    C.  Incorrect: While this is assisted death, so is A, making D the correct answer.

    D.  **Correct**: Both acting to end a patient's life and providing a patient with the medications to end his or her own life are forms of assisted death.

36.    Answer is D

    A.  Incorrect: The patient's report of pain is the most important consideration, not what the family thinks.

    B.  Incorrect: Pain at this level requires immediate action and cannot wait until the next team meeting.

    C.  Incorrect: Always believe what the patient says about their pain. Pain is not always shown in the patient's expression or behavior.

    D.  **Correct**: Increased pain needs immediate attention and should be reported to the RN so that action can be taken.

37. Anorexia is:

 A. Hair loss due to chemotherapy

 B. Abdominal swelling

 C. Loss of appetite

 D. Air hunger

38. Allowing the patient to make their own decisions and respecting those decisions demonstrates which of the following ethical principles?

 A. Beneficence

 B. Nonmaleficence

 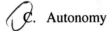 C. Autonomy

 D. Justice

39. Which of the following statements about pain is true?

 A. A large percentage of terminally ill cancer patients and nursing home residents experience pain

 B. The patient's caregiver is the best person to ask about the patient's pain

 C. Patients seldom experience pain during the last days of life

 D. If a patient is able to sleep, she doesn't need pain medication

40. Communication with team members is improved if:

 A. Disagreements are avoided

 B. The team leader always makes the final decision

 C. Roles are strictly enforced

 D. All members are respected for their unique contribution

37. Answer is C

    A. Incorrect: Such hair loss is also known as alopecia.

    B. Incorrect: Such swelling is sometimes called ascites.

    C. **Correct**: Anorexia means loss of appetite. This can be caused by treatments such as chemotherapy or radiation or by the progression of the patient's disease.

    D. Incorrect: Air hunger may be referred to as dyspnea.

38. Answer is C

    A. Incorrect: Beneficence refers to doing what is good for the patient.

    B. Incorrect: Nonmaleficence means not doing anything bad or harmful to the patient.

    C. **Correct**: Autonomy means allowing patient's to make decisions and honoring those decisions.

    D. Incorrect: Justice refers to respect for the moral and legal right of a person.

39. Answer is A

    A. **Correct**: Pain is common among cancer patients and nursing home residents.

    B. Incorrect: The patient is the best person to ask about her pain.

    C. Incorrect: Pain can continue until death. Dying patients still need for their pain to be managed effectively.

    D. Incorrect: A patient may sleep from exhaustion even though the pain is unrelieved.

40. Answer is D

    A. Incorrect: Disagreements, if handled properly, can improve communication and team relationships.

    B. Incorrect: When a team works well together, decision making is shared.

    C. Incorrect: Team members often share roles and learn from other team members how to be effective in various roles.

    D. **Correct**: Mutual respect for each members contribution, skills, and abilities is essential to good communication.

41. Mr. Tingle tells you the doctor told him to take his pain medication every 12 hours and it is working well. Based on this information, you know that:

    A. He is taking the medication wrong and needs to take it more frequently

    B. His pain cannot be relieved unless he takes medication more often

    C. He is on long-acting pain medication

    D. He is confused

42. Which is **NOT** a side effect of opioids?

    A. Drowsiness

    B. Constipation

    C. Nausea

    D. Bleeding

43. A patient's daughter asks you what you think about telling her mother the truth about her condition. Your best response would be that:

    A. Patients shouldn't be told news that might upset them

    B. Patients should be forced to face the truth about their illness

    C. It is best to be honest with the patient in a kind and sensitive way

    D. The doctor will decide what the patient needs to know

44. You arrive at the Parkers' home to find the family very excited that Mrs. Parker, a hospice patient who has been declining physically, sat up, ate dinner and talked with the family for the first time in several days. In responding to this it is important that you consider that:

    A. It is likely that Mrs. Parker will continue to improve and might be discharged from hospice

    B. She was probably overmedicated for pain prior to this event

    C. Dying patients often have a "final rally" days or hours before death

    D. Mrs. Parker is now probably capable of assisting with her personal care

41. Answer is C

   A. Incorrect: Long-acting medications are taken every 8-12 hours.

   B. Incorrect: The correct dose of a long-acting pain medication can effectively control pain without additional medications.

   C. **Correct:** Long-acting pain medications are frequently taken every 12 hours.

   D. Incorrect: His statement is correct.

42. Answer is D

   A. Incorrect: Drowsiness often occurs for one or two days after a new pain medication is started or the dose is increased.

   B. Incorrect: Constipation is present in most patients on pain medications and requires treatment with an effective bowel protocol.

   C. Incorrect: Many patients started on opioids experience nausea for a few days, but it usually goes away.

   D. **Correct**: Bleeding is not a side effect of opioids. It is a possible side effect of other medications.

43. Answer is C

   A. Incorrect: Patients have a right to know about their physical condition even if the news is not good.

   B. Incorrect: Just as patients have a right to know, they have a right not to be told if they so choose.

   C. **Correct**: Patients should be told what they want to know in a compassionate way.

   D. Incorrect: Being honest and informative with the patient is the role of all care providers and family members.

44. Answer is C

   A. Incorrect: Patients can have periods of improvement but most will continue to decline over time.

   B. Incorrect: Patients usually decline physically because of their disease, not because of medications given to relieve pain.

   C. **Correct**: Many patients seem to have a short period of improvement just prior to dying.

   D. Incorrect: A brief period of improvement does not always indicate the patient is capable of greater independence.

45. Apnea is:

    A. A period of no breathing

    B. Decreased circulation

    C. Loss of appetite

    D. Noisy respirations or breathing

46. The nurse tells you that the patient you will be caring for has a subcutaneous (subQ) infusion for pain medication. You know to observe for:

    A. Redness and puffiness at the site

    B. A red streak running along the site of the vein

    C. Fluid leaking around the site

    D. Both A and C

47. Which of the following statements about culture is **TRUE**?

    A. Culture has little influence on a person's beliefs about health and illness

    B. Stereotyping assists with understanding a person's culture

    C. Once learned a person's culture never changes

    D. Culture helps define roles and responsibilities

48. Mr. Miller is having a difficult time getting on and off the toilet due to back pain. The best option for him would be to:

    A. Use a bed pan

    B. Have a catheter inserted by the nurse

    C. Use diapers

    D. Obtain a raised toilet seat

45. Answer is A

   A. **Correct:** Apnea is a period of no breathing that may be followed by a period of breathing.

   B. Incorrect: Decreased circulation is common as death nears.

   C. Incorrect: Anorexia is loss of appetite.

   D. Incorrect: Noisy respirations may accompany apnea, but is not the same.

46. Answer is D

   A. Incorrect: Redness and puffiness at the site is a sign that the needle should be moved but one other answer is also correct.

   B. Incorrect: SubQ infusions are not running into a vein.

   C. Incorrect: Fluid leaking from the site is a sign that the site should be changed but there is one other correct answer.

   D. **Correct**: Both A and C are correct answers.

47. Answer is D

   A. Incorrect: Culture often influences beliefs about healthcare.

   B. Incorrect: Stereotyping or assuming that all members of a group or culture are the same prevents the understanding of an individual's culture as each person is unique.

   C. Incorrect: Culture is always changing depending on a person's lifestyle, significant others, and changing beliefs.

   D. **Correct**: One's culture influences one's roles and responsibilities.

48. Answer is D

   A. Incorrect: This would make Mr. Miller more dependent.

   B. Incorrect: Again this decreases Mr. Miller's independence and would have a negative effect on his skin.

   C. Incorrect: There is no need to insert a catheter when the patient is continent and able to get up.

   D. **Correct**: This intervention promotes his independence and maintenance of good bowel and bladder habits.

49. Antiemetics are used to treat:

   A. Nausea

   B. Increased secretions

   C. Constipation

   D. Anorexia

50. Mr. Williams has a feeding tube inserted in his abdomen. You know that:

   A. He needs to remain flat on his back

   B. Once healed, you can clean the site with soap and water

   C. Drainage around the site should be reported to the licensed nurse

   D. Both B and C

51. Your patient rates her pain as a 3 on a scale of 0-10. In response to this you:

   A. Call the nurse and report the need for increased medication

   B. Ask her if this is an acceptable pain level for her

   C. Ask if you can do anything to make her more comfortable

   D. Both B and C

52. Mr. Thomas just got home from being hospitalized. The nurse tells you he is weak and will need a bed bath. Your best approach to him would be:

   A. Provide all his personal care to help conserve his energy

   B. Encourage him to take a shower with your assistance

   C. Ask him what kind of bath he would like

   D. Ask him if he would like to do any part of the bed bath by himself

49.    Answer is A

    A.  **Correct**: Antiemetics are used for nausea.

    B.  Incorrect: Antiemetics are not used for increased secretions.

    C.  Incorrect: Antiemetics are not used for constipation.

    D.  Incorrect: Antiemetics are not used for anorexia.

50.    Answer is D

    A.  Incorrect: Should have the head of the bed elevated or be sitting upright to prevent aspiration.

    B.  Incorrect: This is a correct answer but so is C.

    C.  Incorrect: This is a correct answer but so is B.

    D.  **Correct**: Once an insertion site is healed, it can be cleaned with soap and water. Drainage around the site should be reported to the nurse.

51.    Answer is D

    A.  Incorrect: A pain level of 3 may be acceptable to the patient and may actually be decreased from previous pain. The nurse should be called if the patient is uncomfortable at their current level of pain.

    B.  Incorrect: You should ask her if she is happy with that level of pain, but there is another correct answer.

    C.  Incorrect: You should ask how to make her more comfortable, but B is also a correct answer.

    D.  **Correct**: Both B and C are actions you should take.

52.    Answer is D

    A.  Incorrect: Allow the patient to determine if he would like to assist with the bath. This promotes a sense of independence and can prevent modesty issues.

    B.  Incorrect: The nurse has ordered a bed bath and you should not take another approach without a changed order.

    C.  Incorrect: Again, you should give the bath as ordered by the nurse.

    D.  **Correct**: This allows Mr. Thomas to maintain some control over his care. He may be more comfortable cleaning parts of his own body if he is able.

53. Which of the following would be a spiritual need of a terminally ill person?

    A. Ask forgiveness from a friend

    B. Tell you her life story

    C. Finish a needlepoint project for her daughter

    D. All of the above are spiritual needs

54. Which of the following statements is **TRUE** about hospice and palliative nursing assistants?

    A. Their role is limited to assisting patients with physical needs

    B. It is not necessary for the nursing assistant to attend team meetings

    C. Their role includes assisting the patient and family in meeting physical, psychosocial, spiritual and emotional needs

    D. Nursing assistant visits to a patient are limited by the Hospice Medicare Benefit

55. Mrs. Kelly asks you why you always exercise her arms and legs when you know she'll never walk again. Your best response would be to say:

    A. "Don't give up hope. You might walk again if you get stronger."

    B. "I'll stop if it hurts you."

    C. "Exercising and using your muscles helps with circulation and keeps your muscles from tightening up."

    D. "Your doctor ordered range of motion exercises."

56. The family of a deceased patient asks you not to touch or clean the body. Your best response would be to:

    A. Tell them it is necessary to prepare the body before the funeral home staff arrives

    B. Ask them to leave the room and proceed with your responsibilities

    C. Recognize that this request could be based on their religious beliefs and practices

    D. All of the above

53. Answer is D

    A. Incorrect: This is a spiritual need but there are other correct answers.

    B. Incorrect: This is a spiritual need but there are other correct answers.

    C. Incorrect: This is a spiritual need but there are other correct answers.

    D. **Correct:** Asking forgiveness, telling one's life story and completing a gift for a loved one can all be spiritual needs of the terminally ill person.

54. Answer is C

    A. Incorrect: The role of the nursing assistant includes more than physical care.

    B. Incorrect: It is very important that the nursing assistant attend team meetings to share observations and participate in care planning.

    C. **Correct**: The role of the nursing assistant includes psychosocial, spiritual and emotional as well as physical assistance.

    D. Incorrect: The Medicare Hospice Benefit allows as many visits as determined necessary by the hospice plan of care for that patient.

55. Answer is C

    A. Incorrect: This might encourage false hope and doesn't address the reason for the exercises.

    B. Incorrect: Range of motion exercises should be continued even if they cause some pain. It might help to give pain medication before the care is provided.

    C. **Correct**: This answers the patient's question by explaining the reason for the exercises.

    D. Incorrect: This is not the main reason for the exercises. Range of motion exercises can also be ordered by the nurse.

56. Answer is C

    A. Incorrect: The family's cultural beliefs and practices should be honored by the hospice team and the funeral home staff.

    B. Incorrect: It is more important to respect the family's beliefs and practices than proceed with the usual tasks.

    C. **Correct**: Several religions require cleaning by specific persons or that the body not be disturbed for a period of time after the death.

    D. Incorrect: Only C is correct.

57. You are very sad about the death of a young patient and can't seem to get him out of your mind. The best action for you to take would be to:

A. Maintain a close relationship with his family to help with your grief

B. Ask that you no longer care for young patients because it upsets you too much

C. Talk with your team members about the death and how it has affected you

D. Try not to get so attached to your patients in the future

58. An adjuvant medication is a medication that is used:

A. For nausea and vomiting

B. To help a patient sleep

C. Instead of pain medication

D. In addition to pain medication to provide more relief

59. Opening windows and having a fan blowing in the room are good initial interventions for:

A. Nausea

B. Breathing difficulties

C. Insomnia

D. Both A and B

60. Culture is:

A. Learned as an adult

B. Learned from a person's family

C. A guide for determining values, beliefs and practices

D. Both B and C

57.    Answer is C

   A.  Incorrect: This is an unhealthy response and an inappropriate professional relationship.

   B.  Incorrect: As a palliative care professional, you need to develop your ability to deal with all types of patients.

   C.  **Correct:** This is a good initial step in getting the support you need. If more help is needed, you need to talk with a professional counselor (such counseling is often available through the organization employing palliative care staff).

   D.  Incorrect: It is only human to feel attachment to the patients, but a professional must learn to set boundaries and take care of him or herself.

58.    Answer is D

   A.  Incorrect: Medications used for nausea and vomiting are called antiemetics.

   B.  Incorrect: Adjuvant drugs may relax a patient but they are not given specifically to help the patient sleep.

   C.  Incorrect: Adjuvant drugs are given in addition to pain medications.

   D.  **Correct**: Adjuvant drugs are given along with pain medication to provide additional relief. Examples are medications for anxiety or depression, anticonvulsants and corticosteroids.

59.    Answer is D

   A.  Incorrect: Opening windows and having a fan blowing are interventions for nausea but another answer is also correct.

   B.  Incorrect: Opening windows and having a fan blowing are interventions for breathing difficulties but A is also correct.

   C.  Incorrect: These interventions are not generally used for insomnia.

   D.  **Correct**: Opening windows and having a fan blowing are good initial interventions for both nausea and breathing difficulties. Therefore A and B are both correct.

60.    Answer is D

   A.  Incorrect: Culture is learned throughout one's life.

   B.  Incorrect: Culture is learned from a person's family but C is also correct.

   C.  Incorrect: Culture is a guide for determining values, beliefs and practices but B is also correct.

   D.  **Correct**: Both B and C are correct.

61. Mr. Lewis, a patient with bone cancer, has some early Stage I skin breakdown. His wife tells you that turning him causes him pain and asks if she can stop. Your best response is to:

   A. Tell her it's okay not to turn him because his comfort is the most important thing

   B. Suggest she turn him after he has had his pain medication

   C. Tell her that turning and repositioning the patient is the best way to prevent further breakdown which may cause him more pain

   D. Both B and C

62. The daughter of a patient who has died invites you to the family's shiva. You know that shiva is:

   A. A meal served for family and friends after the funeral of a Muslim

   B. A Hindu religious ceremony at the grave site

   C. A period of fasting observed by Orthodox Jews

   D. Seven days of intensive mourning observed by Jewish families in their homes

63. A goal of the grief process is to:

   A. Have life be the same as it was before the death

   B. Live successfully without the deceased patient

   C. Replace the deceased person with a new partner or friend

   D. No longer have periods of sadness or crying

61. Answer is D

    A. Incorrect: While his comfort is important, it is important to prevent further skin breakdown which could add to his pain.

    B. Incorrect: This is a good suggestion but not the only correct answer.

    C. Incorrect: This is another correct answer but B is also correct.

    D. **Correct**: Explaining the reason for continued turning and repositioning and suggesting she give pain medication prior to turning are both correct answers.

62. Answer is D

    A. Incorrect: Shiva is a Jewish tradition and not a meal.

    B. Incorrect: Shiva is a Jewish tradition and not a religious ceremony.

    C. Incorrect: Shiva is not a period of fasting.

    D. **Correct**: Shiva is a period of mourning observed by Jewish families.

63. Answer is B

    A. Incorrect: Life will never be exactly the same after a significant loss.

    B. **Correct**: The goal should be to return to a successful life.

    C. Incorrect: New friends and partners are good but should not be made for the purpose of replacing the loved one.

    D. Incorrect: Periods of sadness and crying for the lost loved one may never totally end.

64. Each time you care for Dr. James he wants to tell you about his experiences as a pediatrician. The most important reason for this is that:

A. He wants to impress you with his knowledge

B. He is confused and can only remember past experiences

C. Life review helps a person give meaning and purpose to their life

D. He has no one else to talk to during the day

65. You have tried several times to call or visit a patient's husband to express your sympathy and concern after her death. Your best action now would be to:

A. Document your efforts in the patient's record

B. Write and send a note of sympathy to the patient's husband

C. Report your efforts at the next team meeting

D. All of the above

66. The female patient you are bathing asks you what you think happens after a person dies. Your best response would be to:

A. Tell the patient what your other hospice patients have told you

B. Share your beliefs about life after death

C. Tell her you will ask the chaplain to talk with her about this

D. Ask her to tell you what she believes

67. The most important factor to consider in evaluating a patient's pain is the:

A. Patient's use of pain medications

B. Patient's report about their pain

C. Family's or caregiver's ideas about the patient's pain

D. Patient's diagnosis

64. Answer is C

   A. Incorrect: Reviewing one's life is usually not an attempt to impress another.

   B. Incorrect: Life review is not usually due to confusion.

   C. **Correct**: Life review is an important activity which helps the terminal patient understand and give meaning to his life.

   D. Incorrect: It may be true he has few people to talk to, but this is usually not the reason for life review.

65. Answer is D

   A. Incorrect: Documentation is important but this is not the only correct answer.

   B. Incorrect: It is important to follow up with a note when you are unable to reach the person, but this is not the only correct answer.

   C. Incorrect: This is another important correct action but not the only correct answer.

   D. **Correct**: It is important to document, follow up with a note and report to the team. All of the above answers are correct.

66. Answer is D

   A. Incorrect: It is not helpful to share the stories of other patients.

   B. Incorrect: Sharing your beliefs will not help the patient to explore her own beliefs.

   C. Incorrect: While it would be good to tell the chaplain about the patient's question, putting the patient off is not helpful.

   D. **Correct**: Allow the patient to explore her own beliefs by asking her what she believes. Often patients asking questions like this want to reflect on their own beliefs.

67. Answer is B

   A. Incorrect: The patient's use of medications is important but not the most important factor.

   B. **Correct:** The patient's description of the pain is always the most important factor.

   C. Incorrect: The family's or caregiver's observations can be helpful but they are not the most important factor.

   D. Incorrect: The diagnosis can be helpful information but is not the most important factor in evaluating the pain.

68. You have noticed that your home hospice patient is often laying in urine and feces when you arrive. There are signs that she is not getting her medications or receiving adequate food and fluids. In responding to this situation you know:

   A. It is the social worker's job to evaluate and report abuse and neglect of a patient

   B. The entire team must agree that there is a problem with the care of a patient before it is reported to authorities

   C. Any person who is aware of abuse and neglect has the responsibility of making sure it is reported

   D. What happens to the patient when the team is not present is not the team's responsibility

69. A nursing assistant should check the patient's pain:

   A. If pain management is a problem for that patient

   B. With every visit or patient contact

   C. If the nurse requests such information

   D. Only when the pain medication has been changed or increased

70. Anticipatory grief:

   A. Is more likely to happen if the death is sudden and traumatic

   B. Is only experienced by the patient

   C. Always happens during a long illness

   D. Occurs before the actual death or loss

68.    Answer is C

    A.  Incorrect: While the social worker may assume the primary responsibility for such an evaluation and report, it is the responsibility of any team member observing abuse or neglect to be sure it is reported.

    B.  Incorrect: If anyone believes that a patient has been neglected or abused, that person is responsible for assuring it is reported. Team agreement is not necessary. Waiting for the team to meet may delay mandatory reporting to authorities.

    C.  **Correct**: Anyone aware of a patient's abuse or neglect must report it to the authorities (usually adult protective services).

    D.  Incorrect: The team has responsibility for the protection and safety of the patients assigned regardless of when incidents occur.

69.    Answer is B

    A.  Incorrect: Pain, the fifth vital sign, should be evaluated during each patient contact.

    B.  **Correct**: Pain should be assessed in every patient at every visit.

    C.  Incorrect: Pain should be assessed whether or not the nurse requests an assessment.

    D.  Incorrect: Again, pain should be assessed at every visit.

70.    Answer is D

    A.  Incorrect: Anticipatory grief is more likely to happen when the illness is long and death is expected.

    B.  Incorrect: Anticipatory grief can be experienced by the patient and the family, friends or significant others.

    C.  Incorrect: Anticipatory grief often, but not always, occurs during a long illness.

    D.  **Correct**: Anticipatory grief is grief experienced before the actual death or loss.

71. You are caring for a person of the Muslim faith. You notice that the family has turned the patient's bed and you know this is most likely because:

   A. It is important for the family to be able to get close to the patient for frequent cleaning of the body

   B. The patient must be able to see out a window at all times

   C. The patient's body must face the direction of his holy city at the time of death

   D. All of the above

72. Muscle twitching is a treatable side effect of:

   A. Medication for seizures

   B. Treatment with high doses of opioids

   C. Radiation treatment

   D. Chemotherapy

73. As his death approaches, Mr. Overton's family is very upset by his noisy, rattling respirations. You can tell the family that:

   A. Oxygen will help the patient

   B. The noise is more uncomfortable for them than it is for the patient

   C. Suctioning the patient will help

   D. Nothing will help

74. Fatigue or extreme tiredness in a patient can be caused by:

   A. Diseases and their treatment

   B. Medication side effects

   C. Emotional factors

   D. All of the above

71.    Answer is C

   A.  Incorrect: Although cleanliness is important to the Muslim faith, this would not be a reason for turning the bed in a certain direction.

   B.  Incorrect: This is not required by the Muslim faith.

   C.  **Correct:** When dying, Muslims believe the body should be facing Mecca, their holy city.

   D.  Incorrect: C is the correct answer.

72.    Answer is B

   A.  Incorrect: This is not a usual side effect of seizure medications.

   B.  **Correct**: Treatment with high doses of opioids can cause muscle twitching also called myoclonus.

   C.  Incorrect: Muscle twitching is not a usual side effect of radiation.

   D.  Incorrect: B is the only correct answer.

73.    Answer is B

   A.  Incorrect: Oxygen usually is not helpful for the "death rattle."

   B.  **Correct**: Usually the patient is not suffering or aware of the respirations at this point in time.

   C.  Incorrect: Suctioning is usually not helpful and can be uncomfortable for the patient.

   D.  Incorrect: Repositioning and turning the patient may help and there are medications that can help.

74.    Answer is D

   A.  Incorrect: This is one of three correct answers.

   B.  Incorrect: This is one of three correct answers.

   C.  Incorrect: This is one of three correct answers.

   D.  **Correct:** Diseases and treatment, medication side effects and emotional factors can all be causes of fatigue in patients.

75. In the early stages of grief, it is normal for a person to:

   A. Look for the loved one to return

   B. Deny that the loved one has died

   C. Feel numb and isolated

   D. All of the above

76. Mr. Lane's daughter is visiting when you arrive to do his personal care. Which of the following actions is most appropriate:

   A. Ask his daughter to leave the room during his personal care

   B. Ask Mr. Lane if he wants his daughter to leave during his personal care

   C. Tell his daughter that she can give his bath today

   D. Call the nurse and ask him/her what to do

77. Opioids are:

   A. Narcotics or strong pain medication

   B. Adjuvant medications for pain

   C. Used to treat mild pain

   D. Varicose veins in the rectal area

78. Mr. Overstreet's wife reports that he hasn't had a bowel movement for 3-4 days. He is eating well and remains alert and talkative. While giving his bath, you see he is oozing liquid stool. You:

   A. Tell Mrs. Overstreet that he is trying to have a bowel movement and it should happen soon

   B. Give him an enema

   C. Call the nurse and report that Mr. Overstreet is dying

   D. Call the nurse and report that Mr. Overstreet is oozing stool and may be impacted

75.	Answer is D

    A.	Incorrect: This is one of three correct answers.

    B.	Incorrect: This is one of three correct answers.

    C.	Incorrect: This is one of three correct answers.

    D.	**Correct:** It is normal for persons in the early stage of grief to look for the loved one to return, deny that the loved one has died and feel numb and isolated.

76.	Answer is B

    A.	Incorrect: Mr. Lane might want his daughter to be present and she might want to observe his personal care in order to do it herself later.

    B.	**Correct**: Always ask the patient's permission to have others present during personal care and treatments.

    C.	Incorrect: Never delegate your assigned duties to a patient's family unless they ask to learn and take part.

    D.	Incorrect: There is no need to call the nurse if you handle this properly.

77.	Answer is A

    A.	**Correct**: Opioids are strong pain medications or narcotics.

    B.	Incorrect: Adjuvant medications are not opioids. They are medications used for a variety of reasons including reducing pain.

    C.	Incorrect: Strong pain medications such as opioids are usually started when pain is moderate to severe.

    D.	Incorrect: Varicose veins in the rectal area are hemorrhoids.

78.	Answer is D

    A.	Incorrect: Mr. Overstreet is probably impacted and will not have a bowel movement on his own.

    B.	Incorrect: You should not give an enema without a nurse's order.

    C.	Incorrect: Oozing stool is sometimes a sign that death is near but there is not evidence that this is the case here.

    D.	**Correct**: Call the nurse to report your findings and follow any orders given.

79. Mrs. Anderson tells you she has a durable power of attorney for healthcare. You know this means that:

   A. A lawyer is available to assist her with legal questions

   B. The patient has decided who will get her possessions after death

   C. The patient has named someone to make her healthcare decisions if she cannot

   D. You should ask her husband about any decisions related to her care

80. Your patient's family is present when she dies. The son asks if he can shave his father before the body is taken to the funeral home. Your best response would be to:

   A. Tell him you'll be happy to shave the patient as it is your job to clean the body

   B. Tell him not to worry because the funeral home will do this to prepare the body for viewing

   C. Tell him his father doesn't need a shave

   D. Encourage him to shave his father and offer to assist in any way he would like

81. When people cannot communicate with words, you can evaluate their pain by observing their:

   A. Appetite

   B. Sleep patterns

   C. Relationship with others

   D. All of the above

79.    Answer is C

    A.  Incorrect: Durable power of attorney doesn't refer to an attorney as legal counsel.

    B.  Incorrect: A regular Will (not Living Will) expresses the patient's wishes related to her belongings.

    C.  **Correct**: A durable power of attorney for healthcare appoints someone to make the patient's healthcare decisions when he or she is no longer able.

    D.  Incorrect: While Mrs. Anderson's husband could be her durable power of attorney, it could be another family member or friend, and that person is involved in decision-making only when the patient can no longer make decisions.

80.    Answer is D

    A.  Incorrect: The son probably wants to do this himself as part of his closure with his father.

    B.  Incorrect: Again, the son has other reasons for wanting to do this.

    C.  Incorrect: This ignores the son's desire to do something for his father.

    D.  **Correct**: Always respect the family's wishes related to preparing and handling the patient's body after death.

81.    Answer is D

    A.  Incorrect: Changes in appetite can be a sign of unrelieved pain but B and C are also correct.

    B.  Incorrect: Changes in sleep patterns can be a sign of pain, but A and C are also correct.

    C.  Incorrect: Changes in a person's relationships such as withdrawal or aggressive behavior can be signs of unrelieved pain as are A and B.

    D.  **Correct**: A, B and C are all correct answers.

82.    Which of the following is **NOT** a good statement to use when talking to a grieving family member?

   A.   "I think you should take some time off work to recover from your loss."

   B.   "This must be difficult."

   C.   "How are you handling all this?"

   D.   "What can I do to help you?"

83.    Cheyne-Stokes respirations are most often seen in:

   A.   Patients with lung cancer

   B.   Patients with asthma

   C.   Patients who are actively dying

   D.   A and B

84.    Two of the patients you visit in their homes have gone to the same church for years and know each other well. One day during one of the patients' bath, she asks you how her friend is doing. You respond by:

   A.   Reporting on the status of the other patient

   B.   Telling her to ask the nurse on your team for medical information

   C.   Explaining that you cannot share any information about a patient with any other person without permission

   D.   Explaining that you haven't seen the other patient recently but will give a report the next time you visit

85.    Which of the following is **TRUE** about the grief process?

   A.   All people experience the same feelings and stages

   B.   It begins after the patient's death

   C.   It differs from person to person

   D.   It is easier if the person dying is old

82. Answer is A

    A. **Correct**: You shouldn't give advice to a grieving person.

    B. Incorrect: This is a good statement to make as it shows your concern and opens the door for them to say more.

    C. Incorrect: It is good to ask an open-ended question which allows the person to talk.

    D. Incorrect: It is good to show concern by asking the person what they need.

83. Answer is C

    A. Incorrect: Cheyne-Stokes respirations refers to a pattern of breathing common to a dying patient.

    B. Incorrect: This does not refer to patient with asthma.

    C. **Correct**: Cheyne-Stokes refers to a pattern of breathing in which the patient stops breathing for long periods then suddenly start breathing rapidly.

    D. Incorrect: Cheyne-Stokes respirations occur in patients who are actively dying regardless of their diagnosis.

84. Answer is C

    A. Incorrect: Any information about a patient is confidential and should never be shared with another patient.

    B. Incorrect: No member of the team is allowed to share confidential information without the patient's permission.

    C. **Correct**: You cannot share any confidential information without patient permission.

    D. Incorrect: Again, you cannot share such information and should not make such a promise.

85. Answer is C

    A. Incorrect: Although there are often similar stages to grief, the grief process is different for each person.

    B. Incorrect: The grief process can begin with anticipatory grief long before the patient dies.

    C. **Correct:** Grief is on an individual experience.

    D. Incorrect: A person's grief depends on her relationship and feelings towards the loved one, not her age.

86. Mrs. Summers' family is concerned that she has been sleepy since starting her new pain medication two days ago. In response you:

A. Make sure that Mrs. Summers is responsive when you wake her for her bath

B. Explain to the family that patients are often drowsy when they start a new pain medication but that it usually clears within a few days

C. Follow fall precautions while caring for Mrs. Summers

D. All of the above

87. Each time you care for Mrs. Jackson, she tells you how she wishes she could tell her sister how much she loves her. In response to this, you should:

A. Report her repeated request to the team at their next meeting

B. Ask her questions about her relationship with this sister and listen as she shares

C. Offer to help her write or call her sister

D. All of the above

88. Patients who have had chemotherapy often experience anorexia or loss of appetite. When preparing food for such a patient, helpful actions include:

A. Offer small meals or snacks throughout the day

B. Remind the patient that they must eat to keep up their strength

C. Serve three regular-sized meals as usual to keep the patient on their eating schedule

D. Wait until the patient requests food or fluids

86. Answer is D

    A. Incorrect: Although drowsiness is common when a new pain medication is started, the patient should still be easily aroused and alert when awake. You should monitor this and report your findings to the nurse. Answers B and C are also correct answers.

    B. Incorrect: Sleepiness is common with a new pain medication but usually clears in 1-2 days, but all three answers are correct.

    C. Incorrect: You should always observe fall precautions when patients are on pain medications but A and C are also correct.

    D. **Correct**: A, B, and C are all correct actions to take.

87. Answer is D

    A. Incorrect: This is one of three correct answers.

    B. Incorrect: This is one of three correct answers.

    C. Incorrect: This is one of three correct answers.

    D. **Correct**: Reporting her request to the team, allowing her to discuss her relationship and assisting her to make contact with her sister would all be actions to help Mrs. Jackson.

88. Answer is A

    A. **Correct**: Offering small meals and snacks would allow the patient to eat frequently in small amounts that would not be overwhelming.

    B. Incorrect: While this may be true, it is not helpful to make the patient feel worse about their loss of appetite.

    C. Incorrect: The patient will not be able to eat regular amounts and may feel guilty or bad about refusing food prepared for him or her.

    D. Incorrect: The patient needs food and fluids but may not request any. Offering small amounts and having fluids constantly available is most appropriate.

89. You are caring for a patient with very advanced Alzheimer's disease. On the day of your visit, the patient insists on calling you by her deceased mother's name. The most appropriate action would be to:

A. Remind her repeatedly that you are not her daughter and that her mother is dead

B. Allow her to address you as her mother and respond as you believe her mother would

C. Remind the patient's of the date and year in an effort to orient her to her surroundings

D. Gently tell the patient you are not her mother and acknowledge the importance of her mother to her and her feelings about her mother

90. When communicating with a person who is struggling to express their feelings, you should remember to:

A. Try not to stand in a way that could be seen as towering over him

B. Listen carefully to both the words and the non-verbal things they might be doing (groaning, sighing, etc.)

C. Make sure the person is as comfortable as possible

D. All of the above

91. Delirium is:

A. A state of agitation, restlessness and confusion

B. Insomnia

C. Breathing difficulty

D. Seeing visions or persons not present

89. Answer is D

   A. Incorrect: It is not helpful to correct a person with late stage Alzheimer's disease as they are unable to become oriented.

   B. Incorrect: It is more important to address the feelings behind what she is saying rather than pretend the statements are correct.

   C. Incorrect: Again, it is not possible to reorient a person with advanced Alzheimer's disease.

   D. **Correct**: Speaking gently and acknowledging the patient's feelings is the best response.

90. Answer is D

   A. Incorrect: This is one of three correct answers.

   B. Incorrect: This is one of three correct answers.

   C. Incorrect: This is one of three correct answers.

   D. **Correct**: Sitting so you can look the person in the eyes, listening carefully and observing non-verbal communication, and making sure the person is comfortable are all important actions to take to communicate well. Answers A, B, and C are all correct.

91. Answer is A

   A. **Correct**: Delirium is a state of agitation, restlessness and confusion.

   B. Incorrect: Delirium is not the same as insomnia although delirious patients often have difficulty sleeping.

   C. Incorrect: Breathing difficulty is not delirium.

   D. Incorrect: Delirious persons may see things that are not present, but this is not a definition of delirium.

92. When doing reminiscing with a patient, it is important to:

    A. Allow the patient to do the talking

    B. Change the subject if the patient becomes sad

    C. Give the patient cues about what you want them to talk about

    D. Guide the patient to talk about happy topics

93. When you enter a patient's room in their house, he tells you that he is very angry with his son. Which of the following would be your best response?

    A. "Do you want to talk about it?"

    B. "I can see that you are angry. I'll come back tomorrow."

    C. "Let me let you cool down while I talk to your son."

    D. "Please try not to be angry, I don't want you to get upset."

94. Disenfranchised grief is:

    A. Grief that has lasted longer than one year

    B. Grief that cannot be openly expressed

    C. Postponed grief

    D. When the person feels a physical reaction to a death

92.    Answer is A

    A. **Correct:** Reminiscing should allow the patient to tell their own story.

    B. Incorrect: Some topics when reminisced about may make patient sad. Staff need to be aware that this could happen.

    C. Incorrect: The patient should be allowed to talk about what they want to talk about.

    D. Incorrect: Again, the patient should be allowed to choose the topic, whether it is a happy or sad topic.

93.    Answer is A

    A. **Correct:** Asking the patient if he wants to talk lets him decide if he wants to talk about it or not. You will also want to inform the interdisciplinary team about his anger.

    B. Incorrect: A patient should not be left when angry until you determine that he is okay.

    C. Incorrect: You should talk to the patient first.

    D. Incorrect: Never tell a patient not to feel what they are feeling. Feelings are subjective and therefore are what the patient says they are.

94.    Answer is B

    A. Incorrect: Grief that lasts longer than one year may be abnormal or complicated grief.

    B. **Correct:** Disenfranchised grief happens when the bereaved person's grief isn't accepted by the community. Example could include the loss of a same sex partner or mistress.

    C. Incorrect: Postponed grief may be another example of abnormal or complicated grief.

    D. Incorrect: Physical symptoms like loss of appetite or insomnia are normal reactions to grief.

95. The mother of a 36-year-old woman who has ovarian cancer wants her daughter to have the Sacrament of the Sick, but the daughter is refusing. She tells you that she is Roman Catholic and raised her daughter to be Roman Catholic. Your best intervention would be to:

    A. Call a hospice priest to perform the Sacrament of the Sick

    B. Encourage the daughter to talk to her mother about why she doesn't want the sacrament

    C. Talk to the mother privately to suggest having the sacrament done while her daughter is sleeping

    D. Tell the mother that her daughter has the right to refuse anything

96. Which of the following is **NOT** a sign that death has occurred?

    A. Clenched jaw

    B. Enlarged pupils

    C. Incontinence

    D. Slightly open eyelids

97. While attending the funeral of a patient, you are concerned that a family member is very angry. Your best action is to:

    A. Ask the family member if they would like to talk privately about their anger

    B. Inform the disciplinary team of the family member's anger

    C. Talk to other family members about your concerns

    D. Understand that anger is an accepted part of grieving and no action is required

95. Answer is B

    A. Incorrect: It is not acceptable to call any member of the team to do something that the patient is refusing. You will want to inform the spiritual counselor member of the team of the mother's request.

    B. **Correct:** Different generations may not practice a religion the same way. Encouraging the mother and daughter to talk may give them the opportunity to discuss the differences in their spiritual beliefs.

    C. Incorrect: As long as a patient is refusing something, it is not acceptable to suggest that it be done without their consent.

    D. Incorrect: While the patient does have the right to refuse any treatment, this is not the best way to handle the situation.

96. Answer is A

    A. **Correct:** Initially, following death, the muscles will be relaxed not clenched.

    B. Incorrect: Pupils will be enlarged after death has occurred.

    C. Incorrect: Due to relaxation of muscles, the patient will be incontinent of bowel and bladder.

    D. Incorrect: Though many people will close the eyelids following death, they will be slightly open after death has occurred.

97. Answer is B

    A. Incorrect: Talking about their feelings may assist the family member, but the funeral is not the appropriate place to do this.

    B. **Correct:** Hospice care for the family continues after the death. Letting the team know about the anger will aid them in determining the best approach for this family member. The behaviors you observe will determine when you need to inform the team.

    C. Incorrect: Talking to other family members before someone talks to this family member may be a breach of confidentiality.

    D. Incorrect: While anger can be an expected reaction to grieving, the family member may benefit from some counseling.

98. A patient who is receiving hospice care in her own home that she shares with her daughter. She whispers to you that her daughter is taking her pain medications and asks that you not tell anyone. You have observed that her pain is very poorly controlled. Your response to her would be to:

    A. Ask the daughter if she is taking her mother's pain medication

    B. Assure her that her daughter would not take her medication

    C. Keep her secret, as you do not have proof that the daughter is taking the medications

    D. To tell her that you cannot keep this to yourself as it is hurting her

99. A nursing home patient is experiencing nausea. Which of the following treatments could the nursing home staff try to decrease the patient's nausea?

    A. Add spices to the food

    B. Have a glass of wine before dinner

    C. Placing a warm washcloth on the forehead

    D. Serve food at the patient's desired temperature

100. A patient asks you to assist with a photo album. She also asks you not to tell her family. Your best response is to:

    A. Encourage her to tell her family

    B. Help her with the photo album and tell her family that she does not want them to know what she's doing

    C. Help her with the photo album, do not tell her family, but tell the interdisciplinary team

    D. Tell her you cannot help with the photo album if her family is not aware

98. Answer is D

    A. Incorrect: This is an inappropriate action as the situation needs to be looked into by other members of the team and could produce a violent reaction from her daughter.

    B. Incorrect: You do not know that her daughter would not take her medications.

    C. Incorrect: Whether you have proof or not that her daughter is taking the medication, the suspicion of abuse must be reported.

    D. **Correct:** If the daughter is taking her mother's medication, the mother will not be able to control her pain. This means that the patient is not receiving the care she needs, which may be abuse and must be reported.

99. Answer is D

    A. Incorrect: Spicy food may cause or increase nausea.

    B. Incorrect: Alcohol may cause or increase nausea.

    C. Incorrect: A cool or damp cloth on the forehead is helpful in decreasing nausea, not a warm cloth.

    D. **Correct:** Food served at cool or room temperatures are less likely to cause nausea, but food should be served at the temperature requested by the patient.

100. Answer is C

    A. Incorrect: She has a reason that she does not want her family to know she is working on the album and this should be respected.

    B. Incorrect: You can help her with the photo album, but as the project does not present any harm, her request should be honored.

    C. **Correct:** She has a reason that she wants to work on the photo album without her family knowing which may be part of her own grieving process. The interdisciplinary team will need to know about the project so they can follow up with her to determine if she needs help with an unresolved issue and if the family should be made aware.

    D. Incorrect: She has a right to ask for your help and to do things that her family is not aware of.

# Case Studies
# and Answers

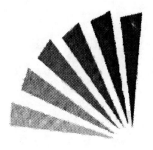

# Case Studies for Discussion

## Case Study #1:

You are caring for an Orthodox Jewish patient who will most likely die before the end of your shift. The family is present in the patient's room. This is your first experience caring for an Orthodox Jewish patient so you are not sure what to expect.

1. Since you are not familiar with Jewish beliefs and practices what would you do?

2. The family requests that the mirrors be covered. Why is this?

3. What might you expect related to handling of the body after death and the burial?

4. Would you expect all Orthodox Jews to follow the same practices and values as this family?

# Case Study #1 Answers

1.  **Answer:** The most appropriate thing to do is ask the family if they have any beliefs or practices related to the care of the dying person that would be important for you to know. Don't assume that because a patient is from a particular religion or culture that the beliefs and practices are exactly the same as others from that culture/religion.

2.  **Answer:** Mirrors are covered because no activity should take place that takes attention away from the person who has died. Looking at oneself in the mirror would distract a person from the person who has died.

3.  **Answer:** After death, the body of an Orthodox Jew is not left alone until burial. The person's eyes should be closed immediately after death, preferably by the deceased person's children. The dead body usually receives a special washing by the Chevra Kadisha, specially trained members of the Jewish community. Orthodox Jews believe burial should take place before sundown of the day following the death. Death is followed by seven days of intensive family mourning called shiva.

4.  **Answer:** It is important to remember that values, beliefs, and practices vary from individual to individual. Health care workers need to avoid making assumptions about people because they are a member of a particular group. Again, the best way to learn about a culture is to ask them or their family what is important to them.

# Case Study #2

Mrs. Casey has advanced Alzheimer's disease. She is still walking. Most of her speech is difficult to understand, but occasionally she responds appropriately. Recently, she has begun pushing food away and is losing weight. Her doctor has done tests and believes that there is no reversible physical problem such as an infection, pain or constipation that might be causing this. The interdisciplinary care team talks to Mrs. Casey's daughter, who is her healthcare proxy (or durable power of attorney for healthcare).

1.  What medical issues should be included in the discussion?

2.  What ethical issues should be included in the discussion?

3.  Mrs. Casey's daughter says that she was told that once the feeding tube is placed, it cannot be removed. What do you tell her?

4.  Is it a good idea to put a tube in and then remove it? Why or why not?

# Case Study #2 Answers

1.   **Answer:** The interdisciplinary care team should talk to Mrs. Casey's daughter about the natural progression of Alzheimer's disease (that is, what happens over a long period of time to the mind and body of someone with this illness) and, in a gentle fashion, what can be expected to happen to Mrs. Casey as her condition worsens. They should also talk to her about what would happen to Mrs. Casey if she has a feeding tube or if she doesn't have a feeding tube. They should also mention that no matter what choice is made as far as treatment, the team will work to keep Mrs. Casey comfortable.

2.   **Answer:** The most important ethical issue is respecting Mrs. Casey's autonomy.   Therefore, a decision should be made based on what Mrs. Casey would have wanted if she could tell us. If Mrs. Casey never discussed this issue, it might help the daughter to think back on her life, her values and what she said about other people in similar situations.

3.   **Answer:** A person who is an appointed healthcare proxy or durable power of attorney for healthcare can make the same decisions as the person herself if she were able. Therefore, she can refuse the tube altogether, or ask to have it removed after is has been put in.

4.   **Answer:** Sometimes, it is a good idea to try a feeding tube for a period of time to see if it helps the person. If it does not help the person, it can be removed. This is called a "time-limited trial." Doing this to try to see if it helps, gives the person making a decision the peace of mind of knowing that they tried everything, even if it didn't work.

# Case Study #3

Mr. Davis is a 90-year-old man who has heart disease and recently had a stroke. He is slightly forgetful, but can still make his own decisions. Mr. Davis has a large family, all of whom visit him regularly. Recently, Mr. Davis' 60-year-old son was killed in a car accident. The rest of Mr. Davis' family wants to keep up a "good front" and does not want him to know about his son's death.

1. What ethical principles need to be applied here?

2. What should the interdisciplinary care team do?

3. What if this case involved bad news about Mr. Davis' condition, such as a diagnosis of terminal cancer, and the family did not want him to be told. What should be done?

As Mr. Davis becomes sicker, he tells you that he is considering taking a "bunch of my pills and ending it all."

4. What is your first response to him?

5. What action should you take after providing his care?

# Case Study #3 Answers

1.  **Answer:** The family may be thinking that they are acting in a beneficent (doing good) manner. However, the ethical principle of veracity (or truth-telling), which is part of the principles of autonomy and beneficence (doing good) should be applied here. The culture in the United States generally demands that a person has the right to the truth, no matter how bad it may be.

2.  **Answer:** The team should explain to the family that the resident has the right to this information. Keeping it from him may be unethical. In addition, he will not understand why his son is no longer visiting him. Most importantly, he will lose the chance to grieve his death with his other family members.

3.  **Answer:** Mr. Davis has the right to be told about his diagnosis. However, this "bad news" does not have to be forced upon him. Members of his interdisciplinary care team should find out from Mr. Davis how much he wants to be told about his situation, and tell him only what he wants to know. Some people would rather not know they have a serious illness. It is the responsibility of the person who is giving this information to find out how much the patient wants to know.

4.  **Answer:** Your first response to a patient's mention of suicide is to explore the statement with him. Ask why he is considering this to be an option. Allow him to express his fears about dying which might include pain, being a burden to others, being alone. Find out if an actual plan for suicide is in place (i.e., patient has a method and has thought through the details). Be a good, supportive listener allowing the patient to explore his thinking behind such a statement. Encourage the patient to seek help related to the problems that are causing him to feel this way. Suggest options for dealing with the fears and factors related to the thoughts of suicide. Never offer to assist or support the patient in a suicide effort: hospice and palliative care offers solutions to the problems that are causing the patient to consider suicide as an option.

5.  **Answer:** After your visit with Mr. Davis you should immediately notify the team of his feelings and your discussion with him. Talk of suicide should never be taken lightly. Mr. Davis needs a complete assessment of his psychosocial condition. All team members need to be aware of his thoughts and feelings and a plan for dealing with his situation needs to be included in his team plan of care.

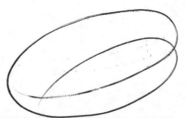

# Case Study #4

Mary Johnson is a 50-year-old female with breast cancer that has spread to her lungs and bones. The report you receive from the team nurse includes the following information: pain is a significant problem for the patient and movement or activity make it worse; the pain medication has recently been increased; the pain has affected the patient's sleep and appetite.

1. You know that you need to check the patient's pain and report back to the team nurse. How would you go about doing this? What questions would you ask? What scales might you use? What would you observe as you provide her care?

2. What non-drug or complimentary treatments might you use while providing care? Describe how to do the treatments you suggest.

3. While providing her care, the patient tells you she is afraid of becoming addicted to her pain medications and is thinking about taking less to avoid this. How do you respond to her?

4. Mrs. Johnson complains that she hasn't had a bowel movement in several days. What do you check related to this problem? What do you do to help the patient with this?

# Case Study #4 Answers

1. **Answer:** You would ask the patient about her pain and observe her as you provide personal care. Questions you might ask her include the following:

   - Where is the pain?
   - How bad is the pain?
   - When does it hurt?
   - How would you describe the pain? (for example, is it crushing, dull, aching, stabbing, pinching, sharp, gnawing?)
   - What makes the pain worse?
   - What makes it better?
   - How does the pain affect other activities such as sleeping, eating, and being with others?

   You would probably ask the patient to rate the pain using a scale. Scales you might use include a number scale, one with faces, one with words to describe the pain, or a pain thermometer. The scale you use is usually the scale everyone in your organization uses to have patients rate their pain.

   While you provide care, you would observe any discomfort the patient has during movement or activity. Sounds the patient makes, facial expressions, changes in breathing, body tension, and the inability to become comfortable are all signs that the patient has pain.

   You should document and report your findings to the team nurse. It is important to report and document everything the patient tells you and all your observations.

2. **Answer:** Non-drug pain management strategies might include distraction, heat or cold applications, massage, imagery, relaxation, music, and aromatherapy. Directions for the various strategies can be found in a variety of reference books.

3. **Answer:** The patient needs to know that addiction is not common in people with chronic pain who are using pain medication as prescribed by a physician to deal with that pain. Fear of addiction is not a good reason to cut back on pain medications. There is no reason for the patient to suffer because of the fear of addiction to the pain medication. You should report this concern to the team nurse so that she or he can discuss it further with the patient.

4. **Answer:** Constipation is a common problem when a patient is taking pain medications. The patient should be asked when her last bowel movement was and the quality of that bowel movement (soft, hard, large or small amount, difficulty in passing, etc.). The patient should be encouraged to follow the bowel protocol as directed by the nurse. You can encourage the patient to be as active as possible, increase her fluids, and eat more fiber if she is eating well. It may help to get the patient up to the toilet if she is bedfast or in the bed most of the time. You should also contact the team nurse to report the constipation and get any related orders.

# Case Study #5

You have provided care for Mr. Dominguez 3 days per week for the past 4 months at his home and are aware of his slowly declining condition. You arrive to give him a bath, and find his family in tears. His wife reports that over the past 24 hours, Mr. Dominguez has been very restless and unable to lie still. He has not been able to sleep, and yet has not been able to communicate clearly with his wife and daughter who have remained awake with him. Mrs. Dominguez states that her husband has been speaking in Tagalog (his first language from the Philippines) and talking about his parents who died many years ago.

1.    What observations do you plan to make, and what will you report to the nurse case manager?

2.    Mr. Dominguez' daughter is fearful that he will get out of bed and fall. She asks whether he should be restrained. What is your response?

3.    What nursing assistant interventions should you begin while in the home?

4.    You find yourself very upset by the changes you see in Mr. Dominguez. You have grown to care deeply for him and his family over the past months. When you get to your car to go home, a feeling of sadness comes over you. What do you do now?

# Case Study #5 Answers

1. **Answer:** Observations and reporting will include: level of orientation, timing of last bowel movement and urination, signs or report of pain, any areas of skin breakdown, shortness of breath, and blue coloring of hands, feet, or lips. You will report statements by the wife regarding Mr. Dominguez' mention of his parents and his use of his primary language. Mr. Dominguez' lack of sleep, ongoing restlessness, and the level of family exhaustion are also important to communicate to the nurse.

2. **Answer:** Provide emotional support to the daughter by acknowledging her concern for the safety of her father. Explain that use of physical restraints is a last resort since they often increase agitation. Suggest ways to make Mr. Dominguez' environment safe, such as placing the mattress on the floor and removing all clutter from the room. Encourage family members and friends to take turns being awake with Mr. Dominguez through the night. Reassure the daughter that you will talk with other members of the interdisciplinary team who will help make plans for the continuing safety and comfort of her father.

3. **Answer:** Provide a calm and comfortable setting by turning off bright lights, turning on soft or familiar music, and offering a soothing bath or gentle massage of the hands or feet. Remain calm, gentle and unhurried in your actions. Suggest that the daughter and wife take a short nap while you are in the home. Make a phone call to the case manager to suggest a visit is needed to further assess and plan for patient and family support.

4. **Answer:** Allow yourself to experience grief and sadness at the loss you are feeling. It is okay to cry or sit quietly for a bit to regain control. You may choose to say goodbye to the patient and family in a formal manner, acknowledging that you may not see them again. If you are feeling overwhelmed, seek assistance immediately; otherwise share your feelings with your team or family upon return to the office or your home.

# Case Study #6

Your 45-year-old female patient is undergoing palliative chemotherapy and radiation for pain and symptom control of her metastatic lung cancer. She tells you she feels "totally exhausted."

1. What are the most likely causes of her fatigue?

2. What are the key observations that you will make and then report?

3. Her family expresses frustration because they think she has "given up." What is your response?

4. List three nursing assistant interventions for the management of fatigue.

# Case Study #6 Answers

1.  **Answer:** Fatigue is a common experience at end of life, affecting 60–90% of cancer patients. There are many reasons for fatigue and it can be difficult to determine one specific cause. In this case fatigue may result from the side effects of current treatments, unrelieved pain, lack of sleep, depression, anemia, or early infection.

2.  **Answer:** You will want to observe for and report changes in behavior or mood, such as tearfulness, decreased appetite, lack of emotion, and decreased social interaction that might indicate depression. It is also important to take vital signs and report elevated temperature or pulse, and to observe the skin for cool temperature or pale color. Any statements that the patient makes about sleep, falls, or family concerns should also be reported.

3.  **Answer:** Reassure the family that there are physical and emotional causes for fatigue. Acknowledge that it is important that the patient participate in activities of daily living and make decisions and choices about her care whenever possible. However, it is likely she will need extra time to accomplish tasks as well as frequent rest periods. Suggest family members use humor and praise to encourage the patient, and avoid criticism or blame.

4.  **Answer:**

    *   Place frequently used items within easy reach, for instance, portable telephone, reading material, tissues, and a glass of water;
    *   Decrease the risk of falls by removing any items along the path to the bathroom, removing throw rugs, and making certain the patient has a way of calling for help;
    *   Encourage activities that help to restore energy, such as meditation, being read to, going out-of-doors, or spending time with pets;
    *   Support independence and decision-making allowing the patient to determine what she is able and desires to do.

# Case Study #7

You have been assigned to care for Mr. West, a 70-year-old man with terminal pancreatic cancer. He has lost his appetite and is eating very little, but his family is still trying to feed him. The nurse has explained to the family that the patient's disease process has caused the loss of appetite.

1.  Why might food and feeding the patient be so important to this family?

2.  How can you help this patient and family with food-related issues?

Mr. West continues to decline and is now approaching death and is too weak to eat or swallow liquids.

3.  What nursing assistant interventions are now appropriate?

4.  What do you now teach the family?

# Case Study #7 Answers

1. **Answer:** Food is associated with living and is a source of comfort. People use food to show their love and concern for others. The family may feel that not providing food is cruel and that the patient will suffer from hunger or starve to death. The patient not eating is also another sign to the family that he is dying and they may falsely hope that if the patient eats, he will get stronger and better.

2. **Answer:** You can reinforce the nurse's teaching about the disease process and the fact that the loss of appetite is due to the disease. The patient's body can no longer use food as it once did. Forcing food can cause the patient to have nausea, vomiting, constipation or bloating and/or diarrhea. Encourage the family to offer small amounts of food and fluids but not to make the patient feel bad if he can't or won't eat. Suggest other ways that they can show their love and concern to the patient such as watching a movie or looking at photo albums, giving him a massage, or talking about favorite memories.

3. **Answer:** Good oral care is extremely important when the patient can no longer take fluids. A toothette or swab can be used to clean out the mouth. A mixture of half water and half hydrogen peroxide can be used to remove dried, crusty secretions. A cool, damp rag can be applied to the face and lips. Vaseline or other lubricating lip treatment can be applied to keep the lips moist. Sometimes, small amounts of water can be put into the mouth using a dropper or syringe, but take care not to put so much that the patient might choke.

4. **Answer:** Teach the family to do good oral care. Reinforce the nurse's teaching about the signs of approaching death. Encourage them to be with the patient and to continue talking with him and expressing their love. Tell them that patients do not suffer from starvation or dehydration at the end of life, but rather this is a natural process of the body shutting down.

# Case Study #8

You are assigned to care for Ms. Greathouse, a young school teacher with melanoma (skin cancer) that has spread to her lungs. She is depressed and often seems to be very angry with those who provide her care.

1. What does the fact that she is angry and depressed tell you about her acceptance of her illness?

2. While you are caring for her, she begins telling you how angry she is at her family and friends. What communication skills should you use as you listen?

3. After she expresses her feelings, Ms. Greathouse asks what you think. How do you respond?

4. The next time you provide care for Ms. Greathouse, she has very little to say to you. How do you respond to this?

# Case Study # 8 Answers

1. **Answer:** Anger and depression are typical responses to loss including the loss of one's health and impending death. It would not be surprising for a young person dealing with a terminal illness to have these feelings. Patients may move on to accept the loss, but not all do.

2. **Answer:** In order to be a good listener, you should focus on the other person. Make eye contact and arrange yourself so that you are at eye level with the patient. Make sure your nonverbal communication says that you are listening to the person. Lean towards the person, nod your head, don't cross your arms and don't appear to be in a hurry. You can ask the person to clarify what they are saying with such comments as "so you mean," or "I understand that you are feeling . . ." Don't interrupt the person. Allow the person to express her anger without making judgments or giving unwanted advice.

3. **Answer:** When you are asked what you think about a situation, don't make judgmental statements or give advice based on your own experience. Repeat what you heard the patient say about her situation and what she wants to do about it. Ask if you have a clear understanding of her feelings and help her to further explore what the best option is for her. Focus on what the patient wants to do about the situation rather than what you think she should do.

4. **Answer:** Silence may mean that the patient is thinking about her situation. Learn to be comfortable with the silence while remaining close and not rushing. Just being present and showing your concern is often helpful to the patient. Ask open-ended questions, but accept it when the patient is not responsive or has little to say. Patients may withdraw after sharing feelings because they are afraid that they will be rejected or that they have revealed negative feelings. The fact that you continue to show care and concern may encourage them to respond.

# Case Study #9

You stop by to visit Mrs. Spalding, the wife of a hospice patient, and express your sympathy several weeks after her husband died. The wife has lost five pounds and has not left the house since the patient's funeral. She tells you that the patient is still talking to her during the night and she says, "I think I'm going crazy."

1.    Are these signs of a normal grief response? Why or why not?

2.    How should you respond to Mrs. Spalding?

3.    What services are available to Mrs. Spalding to help her cope with her grief?

# Case Study #9 Answers

1.  **Answer:** All of these are signs of a normal grief response. Physical responses include loss of appetite, inability to sleep and lack of energy. Bereaved people often withdraw from others. The person is often unable to believe the loss has occurred and may hear the voice of the deceased or think they are present. Often the person experiencing a loss will think they are going crazy as they adjust to such an emotional event.

2.  **Answer:** Your best response is to be a good listener. Learn to be silent and let the bereaved person talk. Respond with a smile, a nod or a gentle touch to let the person know that you understand. Brief statements such as "this must be very hard for you" can encourage the person to share. You should not give advice or say "I know how you feel." Be accepting of the person's thoughts and feelings. You might ask what you can do to help.

3.  **Answer:** Since Mr. Spalding was a hospice patient, Mrs. Spalding will receive bereavement care from the hospice for one year following the patient's death. This might include such services as educational groups on bereavement, support groups, individual counseling, newsletters, memorial services, and social gatherings with other bereaved persons. There are also other community resources such as church-based support groups and widow services. If Mrs. Spalding's grief becomes abnormal or complicated, she may need the services of a professional counselor.

# Case Study #10

Your nursing home patient, Mrs. Parsons, has become totally bedfast due to the spread of her cancer to her bones. The nurse tells you that her bones could break very easily. Due to her lack of movement, skin breakdown could become a serious problem.

1.  What are the causes of skin breakdown in the terminally ill, bedfast patient?

2.  What can you as the nursing assistant do to prevent Mrs. Parsons' skin from breaking down?

3.  What are the first signs of skin breakdown? What actions should you take when you see such signs?

# Case Study #10 Answers

1.  **Answer:** Causes of skin breakdown in the terminally ill bedfast patient include poor nutrition and hydration, immobility, incontinence, circulatory problems, radiation treatments, wound or stoma drainage, certain drug therapies and infrequent repositioning. Poor nutrition and hydration is difficult to change because of the patient's changes in appetite and the weight loss that often goes with terminal illness. Keeping the patient clean and dry can be a challenge when the patient is incontinent, but it's essential to try to keep urine and feces off the skin for any long periods of time. Frequent repositioning of the patient is absolutely essential.

2.  **Answer:** Keeping the patient clean and dry, repositioning the patient at least every two hours, providing range of motion exercises, supporting body parts with pillows, encouraging fluid and food intake when the patient is able to eat, using pressure relieving devices (special mattresses, gel foam pad, heel and elbow pads), avoiding rubbing, pulling or scooting the patient, using a lift sheet to reposition a patient whenever possible are all interventions that the nursing assistant can do to help prevent skin breakdown.

3.  **Answer:** The first sign of skin breakdown is redness in the area of pressure. The red area will blanche or turn white when you apply pressure to it. It is very important to employ techniques such as those listed above at this first sign of skin breakdown.

# GENERAL REFERENCES

Agency for Health Care Policy and Research. *Management of Cancer Pain: Clinical Practice Guidelines.* Rockville, MD: US Department of Health and Human Services; 1994.

Enck RE. The last few days. *The American Journal of Hospice and Palliative Care.* July/August 1992; 11-13.

Fairview Health Services. *The Family Handbook of Hospice Care.* Minneapolis: Fairview Press; 1999

Ferrell BR, Coyle N. eds. *Textbook of Palliative Nursing.* New York: Oxford University Press; 2001.

Frederich ME. Nonpain symptom management. *Primary Care; Clinics in Office Practice.* 2001;28(2):299-316.

Fuzy J. *The Home Health Aide Handbook.* Albuquerque, NM: 2001.

Huang ZB. Nutrition and hydration in terminally ill patients: An update. *Clinics in Geriatric Medicine.* 2000;16(2):313-325.

Kaye P. *Notes on Symptom Control in Hospice and Palliative Care.* Essex Connecticut: Hospice Education Institute; 1992.

Kemp C. *Terminal Illness: A Guide to Nursing Care.* Philadelphia: J.B. Lippincott; 1995.

Kuebler KK, Berry PH, Heidrich, DE. *End-of-Life Care: Clinical Practice Guidelines.* Philadelphia: WB Saunders Co.; 2002.

MacDonald N. Suffering and dying in cancer patients: research frontiers in controlling confusion, cachexia, and dyspnea. *Western Journal of Medicine.* 1995;163(3):278-286.

MacDonald N, Doyle D, Hanks, GWC, eds. *Oxford Textbook of Palliative Medicine.* New York: Oxford University Press; 1996.

O'Brien ME. *Spirituality in Nursing: Standing on Holy Ground.* Boston: Jone and Bartlett; 2000.

Parks C, Laungani P, Young B, eds. *Death and Bereavement Across Cultures.* New York: Routledge; 1997.

Poor B, Poirrer GP, eds. *End-of-Life Nursing Care.* Sudbury, MA: Jones and Bartlett Publishers International; 2001.

Ross DD, Alexander CS. Management of common symptoms in terminally ill patients: Part I. fatigue, anorexia, cachexia, nausea and vomiting. *American Family Physician.* 2001; 64(5):807-814.

Smith SA. *Hospice Concepts; A Guide to Palliative Care in the Terminally Ill.* Champagne, Ill: Research Press; 2000.

Sorrentino SA. The dying person. In Sorrentino SA *Assisting with Patient Care.* St. Louis: Mosby:1999:837-849.

Storey P, Knight C. *Management of Selected Nonpain Symptoms in the Terminally Ill.* Gainesville, FL: American Academy of Hospice and Palliative Medicine; 1996.